RADIANT SKIN

*The Ultimate Guide to Boosting
Your Complexion*

DEVARAJAN PILLAI G

PREFACE

Welcome to "Radiant Skin: The Ultimate Guide to Boosting Your Complexion." In today's fast-paced world, where external stressors, environmental pollutants, and internal factors can wreak havoc on our skin, achieving a luminous and healthy complexion can seem like an elusive goal. However, within the pages of this book, you'll find a comprehensive roadmap to revitalizing your skin and unlocking its natural radiance.

The journey to radiant skin is not just about superficial beauty; it's about fostering a deeper connection with ourselves and nurturing our overall well-being. Our skin is not merely a canvas for makeup or a shield against the elements; it's a reflection of our internal health and vitality. By understanding the intricate balance of factors that influence our complexion, we can embark on a transformative journey towards skin that not only looks good but also feels good.

In this guide, you'll discover a wealth of knowledge distilled from scientific research, holistic practices, and personal anecdotes. From understanding your skin type and identifying common skin concerns to implementing effective skincare routines and making mindful lifestyle choices, each chapter is designed to empower you with practical tools and actionable insights.

Whether you're struggling with acne, hyperpigmentation, or simply seeking to enhance your natural beauty, "Radiant Skin" offers a personalized approach to skincare that celebrates diversity and individuality. We believe that beauty comes in all shades and textures, and our goal is to help you embrace your unique complexion with confidence and pride.

As you embark on this journey towards radiant skin, remember that transformation takes time, patience, and consistency. There may be setbacks along the way, but with dedication and perseverance, you'll gradually uncover the luminosity that lies within.

Thank you for entrusting us with your skincare journey. May this book serve as a guiding light on your path to radiant, glowing skin that radiates from within.

Warmest regards,

DEVARAJAN PILLAI G

COPYRIGHT WARNING

DISCLAIMER

The information provided in "Radiant Skin: The Ultimate Guide to Boosting Your Complexion" is intended for educational and informational purposes only. While every effort has been made to ensure the accuracy and completeness of the content, the authors and publishers make no representations or warranties of any kind, express or implied, about the suitability, reliability, or applicability of the information contained within this book for any particular purpose.

The skincare techniques, recommendations, and advice presented in this book are not intended to replace professional medical advice, diagnosis, or treatment. Readers are encouraged to consult with qualified healthcare professionals or dermatologists before implementing any skincare regimen, especially if they have pre-existing skin conditions, allergies, or sensitivities.

Furthermore, individual results may vary based on factors such as genetics, lifestyle choices, environmental influences, and underlying health conditions. The authors and publishers disclaim any liability for any adverse reactions, injuries, or damages arising from the use or misuse of the information provided in this book.

Readers are advised to perform patch tests and exercise caution when trying new skincare products or procedures, and to discontinue use immediately if any adverse reactions occur. Additionally, the authors and publishers do not endorse any specific brands, products, or services mentioned in this book, and readers are encouraged to conduct their own research and exercise discretion when making purchasing decisions.

By reading this book, readers acknowledge and agree to assume full responsibility for their skincare choices and decisions, and to hold harmless the authors, publishers, and affiliates from any claims, damages, or liabilities arising from such choices and decisions.

Thank you for your understanding.

DEVARAJAN PILLAI G

CONTENTS

1.UNDERSTANDING YOUR SKIN

Types, Textures, and Tones

I n our quest for radiant skin, one of the first steps is to understand the intricate nature of our skin – its types, textures, and tones. Our skin is not only the largest organ of our body but also a complex ecosystem that requires care, attention, and understanding. By unraveling the mysteries of our skin, we can better tailor our skincare routines to achieve the glowing complexion we desire. In this comprehensive guide, we delve deep into the world of skincare to explore the diverse characteristics of different skin types, textures, and tones.

Skin Types

Before embarking on any skincare journey, it's crucial to identify your skin type as it dictates the kind of products and treatments that will work best for you. Broadly speaking, there are four main skin types: normal, oily, dry, and combination.

Normal skin is characterized by balanced sebum production, minimal blemishes, and a smooth texture. It's the holy grail of skin types, often associated with a radiant and youthful complexion.

Oily skin tends to produce excess sebum, leading to a shiny appearance, enlarged pores, and a predisposition to acne and blackheads. Proper cleansing and oil-controlling products are essential for managing this skin type.

Dry skin lacks sufficient moisture, resulting in flakiness, tightness, and rough patches. Hydrating ingredients such as hyaluronic acid and ceramides can help replenish moisture and restore suppleness to dry skin.

Combination skin exhibits characteristics of both oily and dry skin, with an oily T-zone (forehead, nose, and chin) and drier cheeks. Balancing the skin's hydration levels while controlling excess oil in the T-zone is key to caring for combination skin.

Determining your skin type may require some observation and experimentation. Pay attention to how your skin feels throughout the day and how it responds to different skincare products. Once you've identified your skin type, you can tailor your skincare routine accordingly to address its specific needs.

Skin Textures

In addition to skin types, understanding skin textures is essential for achieving smooth and radiant skin. Skin texture refers to the surface characteristics of the skin, including its smoothness, roughness, and pore size. Various factors, such as genetics, aging, environmental damage, and skincare habits, can influence skin texture.

Smooth skin texture is characterized by an even surface, fine pores, and a soft, velvety feel. Achieving smooth skin texture often involves regular exfoliation to remove dead skin cells and promote cell turnover.

Rough skin texture may present as unevenness, bumps, or rough patches, often caused by a buildup of dead skin cells, dehydration, or environmental damage. Gentle exfoliation, hydration, and nourishing skincare ingredients can help improve rough skin texture over time.

Uneven skin texture refers to inconsistencies in the skin's surface, such as fine lines, wrinkles, and visible pores. Aging, sun damage, and collagen loss can contribute to uneven texture, requiring targeted treatments such as retinoids, antioxidants, and collagen-boosting ingredients to improve skin smoothness and elasticity.

Pore size is another aspect of skin texture that many individuals are concerned about. While pore size is largely determined by genetics, factors such as oil production, sun exposure, and aging can affect pore appearance. Regular cleansing, exfoliation, and pore-minimizing products can help reduce the appearance of enlarged pores and refine skin texture.

Understanding your skin's texture allows you to address specific concerns and implement targeted skincare strategies to improve overall skin quality and radiance.

Skin Tones

Skin tone refers to the natural color of your skin, determined by the amount of melanin present in the skin cells. While skin tones vary widely among individuals, they can generally be categorized into several broad groups: fair, light, medium, olive, tan, dark, and deep.

Fair skin tones are characterized by a pale complexion with minimal melanin production, often prone to sunburn and sensitivity. Light skin tones have a slightly warmer undertone and may experience mild to moderate sunburn with prolonged sun exposure.

Medium skin tones range from light beige to olive to caramel hues and are less susceptible to sunburn but still require sun protection to prevent sun damage and premature aging.

Olive skin tones have a greenish or yellowish undertone and tend to tan easily but may still experience sun damage if not adequately protected.

Tan skin tones encompass a wide spectrum of shades, from golden bronze to deep brown, and often have a warm undertone. While tanning may provide some natural sun protection, it's essential to use sunscreen to prevent sun damage and skin cancer.

Dark and deep skin tones have higher levels of melanin, providing natural protection against UV radiation and reducing the risk of sunburn and skin cancer. However, individuals with darker skin tones are still susceptible to hyperpigmentation and other forms of sun damage.

Understanding your skin tone is essential for selecting makeup shades, choosing clothing colors that complement your complexion, and determining the level of sun protection you need. Embracing and celebrating your natural skin tone fosters self-confidence and promotes diversity and inclusivity in beauty standards.

2. THE SCIENCE OF RADIANCE

How Your Skin Works

R adiant skin is not merely a cosmetic aspiration; it's a reflection of the intricate biological processes that occur within our bodies. Understanding the science behind skin radiance is crucial for anyone seeking to achieve a luminous complexion. In this chapter of "Radiant Skin: The Ultimate Guide to Boosting Your Complexion," we delve into the fascinating world of dermatology to explore the inner workings of your skin.

Layers of Protection: The Anatomy of the Skin

Your skin is your body's largest organ, serving as a protective barrier against external threats while regulating temperature and moisture levels. Comprised of three primary layers—the epidermis, dermis, and subcutaneous tissue—each layer plays a unique role in maintaining skin health.

1. The Epidermis: The outermost layer of the skin, the epidermis acts as a shield against environmental aggressors. It consists of several sublayers, including the stratum corneum, which contains keratinocytes that continuously shed and renew to maintain skin integrity.
2. The Dermis: Beneath the epidermis lies the dermis, a dense layer rich in collagen, elastin, and blood vessels. Collagen

provides structural support, while elastin allows the skin to stretch and recoil. The dermis also houses hair follicles, sweat glands, and sebaceous glands, which play vital roles in regulating temperature and moisturizing the skin.

3. Subcutaneous Tissue: Located beneath the dermis, the subcutaneous tissue consists of adipose (fat) cells that provide insulation and cushioning. It also contains blood vessels and nerves that supply nutrients and sensation to the skin.

Cellular Renewal: The Skin's Regenerative Process

Maintaining radiant skin relies on the continuous process of cellular renewal, which occurs primarily in the basal layer of the epidermis. Here, specialized cells called keratinocytes undergo mitosis, dividing to produce new cells that gradually migrate upward through the epidermal layers.

As these cells ascend, they undergo a process known as keratinization, during which they flatten, lose their nuclei, and accumulate keratin—a fibrous protein that strengthens the skin's barrier. Eventually, these fully keratinized cells reach the surface of the skin, where they form the protective stratum corneum.

Understanding this regenerative process is essential for optimizing skincare routines. By supporting cellular turnover through exfoliation and hydration, you can enhance the skin's natural radiance and promote a smoother, more even complexion.

The Role of Moisture and pH Balance

Maintaining optimal moisture levels and pH balance is critical for healthy, radiant skin. The skin's natural moisturizing factors (NMFs), including hyaluronic acid and ceramides, help retain moisture and prevent dehydration. Additionally, the skin's acidic pH (typically between 4.5 and 5.5) serves as a protective barrier against harmful bacteria and environmental pollutants.

Disruptions to the skin's moisture barrier and pH balance can lead to various issues, including dryness, sensitivity, and inflammation. Therefore, incorporating hydrating ingredients and pH-balancing products into your skincare routine can help fortify the skin's barrier and promote a radiant complexion.

The Impact of Lifestyle Factors

Beyond biological processes, lifestyle factors also significantly influence skin radiance. Factors such as diet, hydration, sleep, stress levels, and environmental exposure can all impact the health and appearance of your skin.

1. Diet: Consuming a balanced diet rich in vitamins, minerals, antioxidants, and essential fatty acids can nourish your skin from within. Foods such as fruits, vegetables, lean proteins, and omega-3 fatty acids support cellular function and combat oxidative stress, contributing to a vibrant complexion.
2. Hydration: Adequate hydration is essential for maintaining skin moisture and promoting cellular function. Drinking plenty of water and using hydrating skincare products can help keep your skin plump, supple, and radiant.
3. Sleep: During sleep, the body undergoes crucial repair and regeneration processes, including skin cell turnover and collagen synthesis. Getting sufficient quality sleep allows your skin to rejuvenate, leading to a refreshed and radiant appearance.
4. Stress Management: Chronic stress can trigger inflammatory responses in the body, leading to skin issues such as acne, eczema, and psoriasis. Implementing stress-reduction techniques such as meditation, exercise, and mindfulness can help mitigate these effects and promote skin health.
5. Environmental Protection: Protecting your skin from UV radiation, pollution, and other environmental stressors is essential for preventing premature aging and maintaining a youthful complexion. Incorporating sunscreen, antioxidant-rich skincare products, and protective clothing into your daily routine can help shield your skin from harm.

3.COMMON SKIN CONCERNS

Causes and Solutions

Achieving radiant skin is a universal desire, but it's not always an easy feat. Our skin, being the largest organ of our body, faces a myriad of challenges on a daily basis, from environmental stressors to hormonal fluctuations. In our pursuit of flawless complexion, it's crucial to understand the common skin concerns that many of us encounter and equip ourselves with the knowledge to address them effectively. In this chapter of "Radiant Skin: The Ultimate Guide to Boosting Your Complexion," we delve deep into the causes and solutions for some of the most prevalent skin issues.

Understanding Acne:

Acne, perhaps the most notorious of all skin concerns, affects millions worldwide, regardless of age or gender. It manifests in various forms, including whiteheads, blackheads, papules, pustules, cysts, and nodules. The root cause of acne lies in the hair follicles becoming clogged with oil and dead skin cells, leading to the proliferation of bacteria and subsequent inflammation.

Contributing Factors:

1. Hormonal Imbalance: Fluctuations in hormone levels, particularly during puberty, menstruation, pregnancy, and

menopause, can trigger excessive sebum production, exacerbating acne.
2. Genetics: A family history of acne can predispose individuals to developing the condition.
3. Diet: High glycemic index foods and dairy products have been linked to acne flare-ups in some individuals.
4. Stress: Increased stress levels can stimulate the release of cortisol, a hormone that can worsen acne.
5. Skincare Products: Certain ingredients in skincare and makeup products may clog pores and aggravate acne.

Solutions:

1. Cleansing: Gentle cleansing twice daily helps remove excess oil, dirt, and impurities without stripping the skin's natural moisture.
2. Exfoliation: Regular exfoliation with salicylic acid or alpha hydroxy acids (AHAs) unclogs pores and promotes cell turnover.
3. Topical Treatments: Over-the-counter and prescription treatments containing ingredients like benzoyl peroxide, retinoids, and antibiotics can help reduce acne lesions and inflammation.
4. Lifestyle Modifications: Managing stress through relaxation techniques, adopting a balanced diet, and avoiding pore-clogging skincare products can complement acne treatment efforts.

Addressing Hyperpigmentation:

Hyperpigmentation refers to dark patches or spots that develop on the skin due to an overproduction of melanin, the pigment responsible for skin color. It can result from various factors, including sun exposure, inflammation, hormonal changes, and injury.

Contributing Factors:

1. Sun Exposure: UV radiation stimulates melanocytes, leading to an increase in melanin production and subsequent

hyperpigmentation.

2. Hormonal Changes: Pregnancy, oral contraceptives, and hormonal therapies can trigger melasma, a type of hyperpigmentation.

3. Post-Inflammatory Hyperpigmentation (PIH): Skin trauma, such as acne, burns, or insect bites, can cause PIH, characterized by dark spots at the site of healed lesions.

4. Age: As we age, cumulative sun exposure and slower cell turnover contribute to the development of age spots or liver spots.

Solutions:

1. Sun Protection: Daily application of broad-spectrum sunscreen with a high SPF helps prevent further darkening of existing hyperpigmentation.

2. Topical Agents: Ingredients like hydroquinone, retinoids, vitamin C, niacinamide, and kojic acid are known to inhibit melanin production and fade hyperpigmentation.

3. Chemical Peels: Professional treatments using alpha and beta hydroxy acids or trichloroacetic acid (TCA) exfoliate the skin and reduce pigmentation.

4. Laser Therapy: Various laser and light-based therapies, such as IPL (intense pulsed light) and fractional lasers, target melanin in the skin to lighten hyperpigmentation.

Combating Dryness and Dehydration:

Dryness and dehydration are common skin concerns characterized by a lack of moisture and water content in the skin, respectively. These conditions can lead to discomfort, flakiness, tightness, and premature aging.

Contributing Factors:

1. Environmental Factors: Low humidity, cold temperatures, wind, and central heating can strip the skin of moisture and exacerbate dryness.

2. Aging: As we age, the skin's natural lipid barrier weakens, leading to increased transepidermal water loss (TEWL) and dryness.
3. Harsh Skincare Products: Cleansers, exfoliants, and topical treatments containing alcohol, fragrances, and harsh detergents can disrupt the skin's moisture barrier.
4. Medical Conditions: Eczema, psoriasis, and thyroid disorders are among the medical conditions associated with dry, dehydrated skin.
5. Lifestyle Factors: Smoking, excessive alcohol consumption, and poor dietary choices can impair skin health and exacerbate dryness.

Solutions:

1. Hydration: Drinking an adequate amount of water daily helps maintain skin hydration from within.
2. Moisturization: Applying emollient-rich moisturizers containing humectants like hyaluronic acid and glycerin helps replenish and seal in moisture.
3. Humidifiers: Using a humidifier indoors helps add moisture to the air, preventing excessive skin dryness.
4. Gentle Skincare Products: Opting for fragrance-free, gentle cleansers and avoiding harsh exfoliants and alcohol-based toners can help preserve the skin's natural moisture barrier.
5. Occlusive Agents: Products containing occlusive ingredients like petrolatum, mineral oil, and shea butter create a protective barrier on the skin's surface, preventing moisture loss.

4. CLEANSING 101

The Foundation of Healthy Skin

C lean skin is the canvas upon which a radiant complexion is built. Proper cleansing is not only essential for removing dirt, oil, and impurities but also for preparing the skin to absorb subsequent skincare products effectively. In this chapter of "Radiant Skin: The Ultimate Guide to Boosting Your Complexion," we delve into the fundamentals of cleansing, exploring different techniques, products, and best practices to achieve and maintain healthy, glowing skin.

Understanding the Importance of Cleansing:

Our skin is constantly exposed to environmental pollutants, makeup, excess oil, and sweat, all of which can accumulate on the skin's surface and within the pores. Failure to cleanse effectively can lead to a host of skincare concerns, including acne, dullness, premature aging, and impaired skin barrier function. Cleansing serves as the first line of defense against these challenges, helping to maintain skin health and vitality.

The Benefits of Proper Cleansing:

1. Removal of Impurities: Cleansing eliminates dirt, bacteria, makeup residues, and environmental pollutants, preventing pore congestion and breakouts.
2. Oil Control: Cleansing removes excess sebum, helping to balance oil production and minimize shine.

3. Improved Absorption: Clean skin absorbs skincare products more effectively, maximizing their benefits.
4. Enhanced Skin Renewal: Regular cleansing promotes cell turnover, revealing fresh, radiant skin.
5. Preservation of Skin Barrier: Gentle cleansing preserves the skin's natural moisture barrier, preventing dryness and sensitivity.

Types of Cleansers:

Cleansers come in various forms, each tailored to different skin types and preferences. Understanding the characteristics of different cleansers can help you choose the most suitable option for your skin's needs.

1. Gel Cleansers: Gel cleansers are lightweight and water-based, making them ideal for oily and combination skin types. They effectively remove excess oil and impurities without stripping the skin's natural moisture.
2. Cream Cleansers: Cream cleansers are rich and nourishing, suitable for dry and sensitive skin types. They cleanse the skin gently while providing hydration and comfort.
3. Foam Cleansers: Foam cleansers lather into a rich foam upon contact with water, offering a deep yet gentle cleanse. They are suitable for normal to oily skin types.
4. Micellar Water: Micellar water contains micelles—tiny oil molecules suspended in water—that attract and lift away dirt and makeup without the need for rinsing. It's suitable for all skin types, including sensitive skin.
5. Oil Cleansers: Oil cleansers dissolve makeup, sunscreen, and excess oil, leaving the skin clean and hydrated. They are suitable for all skin types, including oily and acne-prone skin.

Choosing the Right Cleanser:

When selecting a cleanser, consider your skin type, concerns, and preferences. Opt for gentle, fragrance-free formulas that effectively cleanse without causing irritation or stripping the skin's natural oils.

Avoid harsh ingredients like sulfates and alcohol, which can disrupt the skin barrier and cause dryness.

Cleansing Techniques:

The way you cleanse your skin can impact its health and appearance. Follow these techniques to ensure a thorough yet gentle cleanse:

1. Double Cleansing: Start with an oil-based cleanser to remove makeup, sunscreen, and excess oil, followed by a water-based cleanser to remove impurities and sweat.
2. Gentle Massage: Use circular motions to massage the cleanser into the skin, focusing on areas prone to congestion, such as the T-zone.
3. Rinse Thoroughly: Rinse your face with lukewarm water to remove all traces of cleanser, avoiding hot water, which can strip the skin.
4. Pat Dry: Gently pat your skin dry with a clean towel, avoiding rubbing, which can cause irritation.
5. Follow with Toner: After cleansing, apply a gentle, alcohol-free toner to balance the skin's pH and prepare it for subsequent skincare products.

Incorporating Cleansing into Your Skincare Routine:

Consistency is key when it comes to cleansing. Make cleansing a part of your morning and evening skincare routine to maintain a clean, healthy complexion. Follow these steps for optimal results:

Morning Routine:

1. Splash your face with water to refresh the skin.
2. Gently cleanse with a mild cleanser to remove overnight impurities and prepare the skin for the day ahead.
3. Follow with toner, serum, moisturizer, and sunscreen.

Evening Routine:

1. Remove makeup and sunscreen with an oil-based cleanser.

2. Follow with a water-based cleanser to remove remaining impurities.
3. Optionally, use a gentle exfoliator or mask 2-3 times a week to promote cell turnover and reveal radiant skin.
4. Follow with toner, serum, and moisturizer to replenish and hydrate the skin overnight.

5. EXFOLIATION ESSENTIALS

Buffing Away Dullness

Exfoliation is a fundamental step in any skincare routine, playing a crucial role in maintaining healthy, radiant skin. By sloughing away dead skin cells, exfoliation helps unclog pores, smooth the skin's texture, and enhance its natural radiance. In this chapter of "Radiant Skin: The Ultimate Guide to Boosting Your Complexion," we'll delve deep into the essentials of exfoliation, exploring its benefits, different methods, and best practices for achieving optimal results.

Understanding Exfoliation:

Exfoliation is the process of removing dead skin cells from the skin's surface, revealing fresher, more youthful-looking skin underneath. Our skin naturally sheds dead cells as part of its renewal process, but factors such as aging, sun damage, and environmental stressors can disrupt this process, leading to a buildup of dead skin cells and a dull, lackluster complexion.

The Benefits of Exfoliation:

1. Enhanced Skin Texture: Regular exfoliation helps smooth rough, uneven skin texture, leaving it soft and supple to the touch.
2. Improved Skin Tone: By removing dead skin cells, exfoliation promotes cell turnover, leading to a brighter, more even skin

tone.

3. Deep Cleansing: Exfoliation unclogs pores, preventing the buildup of debris, oil, and bacteria that can lead to breakouts and blemishes.
4. Better Product Absorption: By eliminating the barrier of dead skin cells, exfoliation allows skincare products to penetrate more effectively, maximizing their efficacy.
5. Anti-Aging Benefits: Exfoliation stimulates collagen production, helping to reduce the appearance of fine lines, wrinkles, and other signs of aging.

Types of Exfoliation:

1. Physical Exfoliation: Physical exfoliants use abrasive particles or tools to manually scrub away dead skin cells. Common physical exfoliants include scrubs, brushes, loofahs, and microdermabrasion devices.
2. Chemical Exfoliation: Chemical exfoliants use acids or enzymes to dissolve the bonds between dead skin cells, facilitating their removal. Common chemical exfoliants include alpha hydroxy acids (AHAs) such as glycolic acid and lactic acid, beta hydroxy acids (BHAs) such as salicylic acid, and fruit enzymes such as papain and bromelain.

Best Practices for Exfoliation:

1. Know Your Skin Type: Different skin types have different exfoliation needs. Those with sensitive or dry skin should opt for gentler exfoliants, while those with oily or acne-prone skin may benefit from more potent exfoliating agents.
2. Start Slow: If you're new to exfoliation or trying a new product, start with a lower concentration or frequency to avoid irritation or over-exfoliation.
3. Patch Test: Before applying any exfoliant to your face, perform a patch test on a small area of skin to check for any adverse reactions.

4. Follow Instructions: Always follow the manufacturer's instructions when using exfoliating products, including recommended usage frequency and duration of application.
5. Protect Your Skin: After exfoliating, follow up with a hydrating moisturizer and broad-spectrum sunscreen to protect your skin from moisture loss and sun damage.

DIY Exfoliation Recipes:

1. Sugar Scrub: Mix together equal parts sugar and coconut oil to create a gentle scrub that buffs away dead skin cells while moisturizing the skin.
2. Yogurt Mask: Combine plain yogurt with a teaspoon of honey and a squeeze of lemon juice. Apply to the face and leave on for 10-15 minutes before rinsing off to reveal smoother, brighter skin.
3. Oatmeal Scrub: Grind oatmeal into a fine powder and mix with water to form a paste. Massage onto damp skin in circular motions, then rinse off for a gentle exfoliating experience.

Professional Exfoliation Treatments:

1. Microdermabrasion: A non-invasive procedure that uses a diamond-tipped wand or crystals to exfoliate the skin, revealing smoother, more radiant skin underneath.
2. Chemical Peels: A chemical solution is applied to the skin to exfoliate the outer layers, leading to improved texture, tone, and clarity. Chemical peels can vary in strength, from superficial to deep, depending on the desired results and skin type.

6.HYDRATION HACKS

Nourishing Your Skin from Within

Hydration is the cornerstone of healthy, radiant skin. Just as water is essential for sustaining life, it plays a critical role in maintaining the health and vitality of our skin. In this chapter of "Radiant Skin: The Ultimate Guide to Boosting Your Complexion," we delve into the importance of hydration and explore effective strategies for nourishing your skin from within. From understanding the science behind skin hydration to practical tips for maintaining optimal moisture levels, let's embark on a journey to unlock the secrets of hydrated, glowing skin.

The Science of Skin Hydration:

Before delving into hydration hacks, it's essential to understand the underlying mechanisms of skin hydration. Our skin consists of three primary layers: the epidermis, dermis, and subcutaneous tissue. The epidermis, the outermost layer, acts as a protective barrier against external aggressors, while the dermis contains essential structures like blood vessels, nerves, and collagen fibers. Both layers play pivotal roles in maintaining skin hydration.

The epidermis contains specialized cells called keratinocytes, which produce a lipid-rich substance known as the stratum corneum. This outermost layer of the epidermis acts as a barrier that prevents water loss from the skin and protects against environmental stressors. Within the stratum corneum, natural moisturizing factors (NMFs) like amino acids, urea, and lactic acid help attract and retain moisture, maintaining optimal hydration levels.

In the dermis, fibroblasts produce collagen and elastin, proteins that provide structural support and elasticity to the skin. Hyaluronic acid, a naturally occurring molecule found in the dermis, plays a crucial role in maintaining skin hydration by binding water molecules and promoting tissue hydration.

Factors Affecting Skin Hydration:

Several internal and external factors can impact skin hydration levels, leading to dryness, dullness, and premature aging. Understanding these factors is key to developing an effective hydration strategy.

1. Environmental Factors: Exposure to harsh weather conditions, such as cold temperatures, wind, and low humidity, can strip the skin of its natural oils and moisture, leading to dehydration.
2. Lifestyle Habits: Poor dietary choices, inadequate water intake, smoking, and excessive alcohol consumption can impair skin health and contribute to dehydration.
3. Age: As we age, the skin's ability to retain moisture diminishes due to a decline in the production of essential proteins like collagen and hyaluronic acid.
4. Skincare Products: Harsh cleansers, exfoliants, and topical treatments containing alcohol or fragrances can disrupt the skin's natural moisture barrier, leading to dehydration.
5. Medical Conditions: Certain medical conditions, such as eczema, psoriasis, and thyroid disorders, can compromise the skin's ability to retain moisture, resulting in dryness and dehydration.

Hydration Hacks for Healthy Skin:

Now that we've explored the science behind skin hydration and identified factors that can affect moisture levels, let's delve into practical hydration hacks to nourish your skin from within:

1. Stay Hydrated: The most fundamental hydration hack is to drink an adequate amount of water throughout the day. Aim for at least eight glasses of water daily, and increase your intake during hot weather or strenuous physical activity.

2. Eat Water-Rich Foods: Incorporate hydrating foods like fruits and vegetables into your diet. Cucumber, watermelon, oranges, strawberries, and leafy greens are excellent choices, as they contain high water content and essential vitamins and minerals that promote skin health.

3. Hydration Supplements: Consider adding supplements like hyaluronic acid or collagen peptides to your daily regimen. These supplements can support skin hydration from within and improve skin elasticity and texture over time.

4. Use Humidifiers: Invest in a humidifier for your home or office to add moisture to the air, especially during dry winter months. This helps prevent excessive moisture loss from the skin and maintains a comfortable indoor environment.

5. Limit Alcohol and Caffeine: Both alcohol and caffeine can have dehydrating effects on the body. Limit your consumption of alcoholic and caffeinated beverages, and opt for hydrating alternatives like herbal teas or infused water.

6. Choose Hydrating Skincare Products: Look for skincare products formulated with hydrating ingredients like hyaluronic acid, glycerin, ceramides, and natural oils. These ingredients help replenish moisture, strengthen the skin's barrier, and lock in hydration.

7. Moisturize Regularly: Incorporate a hydrating moisturizer into your daily skincare routine, applying it morning and night to clean, damp skin. Choose a moisturizer suited to your skin type, whether it's lightweight for oily skin or rich and emollient for dry skin.

8. Protect Your Skin: Apply a broad-spectrum sunscreen with SPF 30 or higher every day, even on cloudy days. Sunscreen helps prevent UV-induced damage, which can lead to dehydration, premature aging, and skin cancer.

9. Practice Gentle Cleansing: Avoid harsh cleansers that strip the skin of its natural oils and disrupt its moisture barrier. Opt for gentle, hydrating cleansers that cleanse effectively without leaving the skin feeling tight or dry.

10. Hydrating Masks and Treatments: Treat your skin to hydrating masks and treatments once or twice a week to replenish moisture and revive dull, dehydrated skin. Look for products containing ingredients like hyaluronic acid, aloe vera, honey, and botanical extracts.

7.SUN PROTECTION SECRETS

Shielding Your Skin from Harmful Rays

In the pursuit of radiant skin, there's one essential step that often gets overlooked: sun protection. While the sun provides warmth and light essential for life, its ultraviolet (UV) rays can wreak havoc on our skin, leading to premature aging, sunburns, and even skin cancer. In this chapter of "Radiant Skin: The Ultimate Guide to Boosting Your Complexion," we delve into the importance of sun protection, the science behind UV radiation, and effective strategies for safeguarding your skin from the sun's harmful rays.

Understanding UV Radiation:

Before delving into sun protection strategies, it's crucial to understand the two primary types of UV radiation emitted by the sun: UVA and UVB.

1. UVA Rays: UVA rays penetrate deep into the skin's dermis, causing long-term damage such as premature aging, wrinkles, and loss of elasticity. They are also responsible for tanning.
2. UVB Rays: UVB rays primarily affect the skin's outermost layer, the epidermis, and are the primary cause of sunburns. Prolonged exposure to UVB rays increases the risk of skin cancer.

Both UVA and UVB rays can contribute to the development of skin cancer, including melanoma, the deadliest form of skin cancer. Additionally, UV radiation can suppress the immune system, making the skin more susceptible to infections and other environmental damage.

The Importance of Sun Protection:

Given the harmful effects of UV radiation, sun protection is paramount for maintaining healthy, radiant skin. Incorporating sun protection measures into your daily skincare routine not only helps prevent sunburns and premature aging but also reduces the risk of skin cancer.

1. Sunburn Prevention: Sunburns not only cause discomfort but also indicate skin damage. By applying sunscreen regularly and seeking shade during peak sun hours, you can minimize the risk of sunburns and protect your skin from immediate harm.
2. Anti-Aging Benefits: Sun exposure is one of the leading causes of premature aging, including wrinkles, fine lines, and age spots. By shielding your skin from UV radiation, you can maintain a youthful complexion and delay the signs of aging.
3. Skin Cancer Prevention: Skin cancer rates continue to rise globally, making sun protection a critical component of skin cancer prevention efforts. By reducing UV exposure through sunscreen, protective clothing, and seeking shade, you can lower your risk of developing skin cancer.

Sun Protection Strategies:

1. Broad-Spectrum Sunscreen: Choose a broad-spectrum sunscreen with SPF 30 or higher that protects against both UVA and UVB rays. Apply sunscreen generously to all exposed skin areas at least 15 minutes before sun exposure, and reapply every two hours or immediately after swimming or sweating.
2. Protective Clothing: Wear lightweight, long-sleeved shirts, pants, and wide-brimmed hats to shield your skin from direct

sun exposure. Consider clothing with built-in UPF (Ultraviolet Protection Factor) for added sun protection.

3. Sunglasses: Protect your eyes from UV radiation by wearing sunglasses that block 100% of UVA and UVB rays. Look for sunglasses labeled as UV400 or offer 100% UV protection.

4. Seek Shade: Limit sun exposure during peak hours, typically between 10 a.m. and 4 p.m., when UV radiation is strongest. Take breaks in shaded areas or use umbrellas or canopies to create shade outdoors.

5. Avoid Tanning Beds: Tanning beds emit harmful UV radiation that can increase the risk of skin cancer and accelerate skin aging. Opt for safer alternatives like self-tanning products or spray tans for a bronzed glow.

The Role of Antioxidants:

In addition to external sun protection measures, incorporating antioxidants into your skincare routine can provide added protection against UV-induced damage. Antioxidants such as vitamin C, vitamin E, and green tea extract neutralize free radicals generated by UV radiation, helping to prevent oxidative stress and DNA damage in the skin.

8.SERUMS, ESSENCES, AND AMPOULES

Targeted Treatments for Every Concern

I n the quest for radiant skin, a basic skincare routine may not always suffice. While cleansers and moisturizers are essential, sometimes our skin requires targeted treatments to address specific concerns effectively. This is where serums, essences, and ampoules come into play. These concentrated formulations are designed to deliver potent ingredients deep into the skin, targeting everything from fine lines and wrinkles to hyperpigmentation and dehydration. In this chapter of "Radiant Skin: The Ultimate Guide to Boosting Your Complexion," we delve into the world of serums, essences, and ampoules, exploring their unique benefits and how they can transform your skincare routine.

Understanding Serums, Essences, and Ampoules:

Before we delve into the specifics of each treatment, let's define what sets serums, essences, and ampoules apart from traditional skincare products.

1. Serums: Serums are lightweight, fast-absorbing formulations packed with high concentrations of active ingredients. They typically have a liquid or gel-like consistency and are designed to target specific skincare concerns, such as wrinkles, dark spots, or hydration.

2. Essences: Essences are similar to serums but are slightly more viscous and often contain a higher water content. They serve as a hydration booster, helping to replenish moisture levels in the skin and prepare it to better absorb subsequent skincare products.
3. Ampoules: Ampoules are supercharged serums with an even higher concentration of active ingredients. They often come in small, single-use vials or capsules and are intended for short-term use as an intensive treatment to address specific skin concerns.

The key difference between these formulations lies in their consistency and concentration of active ingredients. While serums and ampoules are highly concentrated and target-specific concerns, essences focus primarily on hydration and skin conditioning.

Benefits of Serums, Essences, and Ampoules:

1. High Potency: Thanks to their concentrated formulations, serums, essences, and ampoules deliver a potent dose of active ingredients deep into the skin, providing faster and more noticeable results.
2. Targeted Treatment: Each formulation is designed to address specific skincare concerns, whether it's fine lines, dark spots, acne, or dehydration. This targeted approach allows for a more tailored skincare regimen.
3. Lightweight Texture: Unlike heavy creams or lotions, serums, essences, and ampoules have lightweight textures that absorb quickly into the skin, making them suitable for layering and suitable for all skin types, including oily and acne-prone skin.
4. Enhanced Absorption: These formulations penetrate the skin's barrier more effectively, allowing for better absorption of active ingredients and maximizing their efficacy.
5. Versatility: Serums, essences, and ampoules can be easily incorporated into existing skincare routines, either as standalone treatments or layered underneath moisturizers and sunscreens.

Choosing the Right Formulation:

With a plethora of serums, essences, and ampoules available on the market, choosing the right formulation can be overwhelming. Here are some factors to consider when selecting the best treatment for your skin concerns:

1. Ingredients: Look for formulations containing ingredients that target your specific skincare concerns. For example, vitamin C serums are excellent for brightening and evening out skin tone, while hyaluronic acid serums are ideal for hydration.
2. Skin Type: Consider your skin type and concerns when choosing a formulation. Those with oily or acne-prone skin may benefit from lightweight, oil-free serums, while those with dry or sensitive skin may prefer hydrating essences or soothing ampoules.
3. Texture and Consistency: Pay attention to the texture and consistency of the product. Serums are typically lightweight and fast-absorbing, while essences may have a slightly thicker texture. Ampoules are often more concentrated and may feel slightly heavier on the skin.
4. Packaging: Consider the packaging of the product, especially for ampoules, which often come in single-use vials. Look for formulations with airtight packaging or opaque bottles to protect the ingredients from oxidation and degradation.

Incorporating Serums, Essences, and Ampoules into Your Skincare Routine:

Now that you understand the benefits of serums, essences, and ampoules let's discuss how to incorporate them into your skincare routine effectively.

1. Cleanse: Start by cleansing your skin to remove dirt, oil, and impurities. Choose a gentle cleanser that won't strip the skin of its natural oils.
2. Tone: Follow up with a hydrating toner to balance the skin's pH levels and prepare it to better absorb subsequent skincare products.

3. Treat: Apply your chosen serum, essence, or ampoule to target specific skincare concerns. Dispense a small amount onto your fingertips and gently pat it into the skin until fully absorbed.
4. Moisturize: Follow up with a moisturizer to seal in hydration and provide additional nourishment to the skin. Choose a moisturizer suitable for your skin type and concerns.
5. Protect: Finish your skincare routine with a broad-spectrum sunscreen to protect your skin from UV damage and prevent premature aging.

Remember to patch test new products before incorporating them into your routine, especially if you have sensitive skin or allergies. Start by using the product every other day to assess how your skin responds, and gradually increase frequency as needed.

Common Ingredients in Serums, Essences, and Ampoules:

1. Hyaluronic Acid: Known for its hydrating properties, hyaluronic acid attracts and retains moisture in the skin, helping to plump and smooth fine lines and wrinkles.
2. Vitamin C: A potent antioxidant, vitamin C brightens the skin, evens out skin tone, and protects against environmental damage.
3. Retinol: A derivative of vitamin A, retinol stimulates cell turnover, reduces the appearance of fine lines and wrinkles, and improves overall skin texture.
4. Niacinamide: Also known as vitamin B3, niacinamide helps reduce inflammation, minimize pores, and regulate sebum production, making it ideal for oily and acne-prone skin.
5. Peptides: Peptides are amino acids that help stimulate collagen production, improve skin elasticity, and reduce the signs of aging.

9. THE POWER OF MOISTURIZATION

Hydrating for a Youthful Glow

Moisturization is the cornerstone of any effective skincare routine, serving as a vital step in achieving and maintaining radiant, healthy skin. Our skin is exposed to a myriad of environmental stressors daily, from harsh weather conditions to pollution and UV radiation. These factors can strip the skin of its natural moisture, leading to dryness, dullness, and premature aging. In this chapter of "Radiant Skin: The Ultimate Guide to Boosting Your Complexion," we explore the transformative power of moisturization and how it contributes to a youthful, glowing complexion.

Understanding the Skin's Moisture Barrier:

Before delving into the benefits of moisturization, it's essential to understand the skin's natural moisture barrier, also known as the stratum corneum. This outermost layer of the epidermis plays a crucial role in maintaining optimal hydration levels and protecting the skin from external aggressors.

The stratum corneum consists of dead skin cells embedded in a matrix of lipids, including ceramides, cholesterol, and fatty acids. This lipid barrier acts as a protective shield, preventing water loss from the skin and maintaining its suppleness and elasticity.

However, various factors, such as age, environmental stressors, and improper skincare practices, can compromise the skin's moisture barrier, leading to dehydration and skin conditions like dryness, flakiness, and sensitivity.

The Benefits of Moisturization:

Moisturization replenishes the skin's moisture levels, strengthens its natural barrier, and promotes overall skin health. By incorporating moisturizers into your skincare routine, you can enjoy a myriad of benefits, including:

1. Hydration: Moisturizers deliver essential hydration to the skin, restoring moisture lost due to environmental factors, cleansing, and exfoliation. Hydrated skin appears plump, smooth, and youthful, with a natural radiance.
2. Barrier Repair: Moisturizers containing occlusive and humectant ingredients help repair and strengthen the skin's natural barrier, preventing moisture loss and enhancing its ability to retain water. This, in turn, improves skin texture and resilience, reducing the risk of dryness, irritation, and inflammation.
3. Anti-Aging Effects: Properly moisturized skin appears more youthful and vibrant, as hydration helps minimize the appearance of fine lines, wrinkles, and other signs of aging. Moisturizers containing antioxidants and anti-aging ingredients further protect the skin from environmental damage and promote collagen production, resulting in firmer, smoother skin over time.
4. Protection: Some moisturizers contain SPF (Sun Protection Factor) to provide additional protection against harmful UV radiation, reducing the risk of sunburns, premature aging, and skin cancer. Daily use of moisturizers with sunscreen helps shield the skin from UV-induced damage and maintains its health and vitality.

Types of Moisturizers:

Moisturizers come in various forms, including creams, lotions, gels, serums, and oils, each tailored to different skin types and concerns. Understanding the characteristics of each type can help you choose the most suitable moisturizer for your skin's needs:

1. Creams: Creams are thick, emollient-rich formulations ideal for dry or mature skin types. They provide intense hydration and create a protective barrier on the skin's surface, sealing in moisture and preventing water loss.
2. Lotions: Lotions are lighter in texture than creams and are suitable for normal to combination skin types. They absorb quickly into the skin, delivering hydration without feeling heavy or greasy.
3. Gels: Gels are lightweight, water-based formulations ideal for oily or acne-prone skin. They provide hydration without clogging pores, making them suitable for individuals with sensitive or acne-prone skin.
4. Serums: Serums are concentrated formulations containing active ingredients like hyaluronic acid, vitamins, and antioxidants. They penetrate deeply into the skin, delivering targeted hydration and addressing specific skin concerns like dullness, fine lines, and uneven texture.
5. Oils: Facial oils are rich in nourishing fatty acids and antioxidants, providing intense hydration and improving skin elasticity. They are particularly beneficial for dry or mature skin types and can be used alone or layered over moisturizers for added hydration and glow.

Choosing the Right Moisturizer:

Selecting the right moisturizer for your skin type and concerns is essential for achieving optimal results. Consider the following factors when choosing a moisturizer:

1. Skin Type: Determine whether your skin is dry, oily, combination, or sensitive, and choose a moisturizer formulated to address your specific needs.

2. Ingredients: Look for moisturizers containing hydrating ingredients like hyaluronic acid, glycerin, and ceramides, as well as antioxidants and anti-aging compounds for added benefits.
3. Texture: Choose a moisturizer with a texture that suits your preferences and skin type, whether it's a lightweight gel, creamy lotion, or rich cream.
4. SPF: If you spend time outdoors, opt for a moisturizer with built-in SPF to protect your skin from UV radiation and prevent sun damage.

Incorporating Moisturization into Your Skincare Routine:

To reap the full benefits of moisturization, it's essential to incorporate it into your daily skincare routine. Follow these steps for optimal hydration and a radiant complexion:

1. Cleanse: Start by cleansing your skin with a gentle, hydrating cleanser to remove dirt, oil, and impurities without stripping away moisture.
2. Exfoliate: Exfoliate your skin regularly to slough off dead skin cells and promote cell turnover, allowing moisturizers to penetrate more effectively.
3. Apply Moisturizer: Dispense a small amount of moisturizer onto your fingertips and gently massage it into your skin using upward and outward motions. Pay attention to areas prone to dryness, such as the cheeks, forehead, and neck.
4. Layer Serums: If using serums or treatment products, apply them before your moisturizer to ensure maximum absorption and efficacy.
5. Protect: Finish your skincare routine by applying a broad-spectrum sunscreen with SPF 30 or higher to shield your skin from harmful UV radiation and prevent sun damage.

10. ACNE DEMYSTIFIED

Strategies for Clearing Up Troublesome Skin

Acne, a common skin condition characterized by pimples, blackheads, and whiteheads, affects millions of people worldwide, regardless of age, gender, or ethnicity. Often associated with adolescence, acne can persist into adulthood and pose significant challenges to self-esteem and confidence. In this chapter of "Radiant Skin: The Ultimate Guide to Boosting Your Complexion," we delve into the causes, types, and effective strategies for managing acne and achieving clear, blemish-free skin.

Understanding Acne:

Acne occurs when hair follicles become clogged with oil and dead skin cells, leading to the formation of comedones (non-inflammatory lesions) and inflammatory lesions such as papules, pustules, nodules, and cysts. Several factors contribute to the development of acne, including:

1. Excess Sebum Production: Hormonal changes during puberty, menstruation, pregnancy, and stress can stimulate the sebaceous glands to produce more oil (sebum), leading to clogged pores and acne breakouts.
2. Bacterial Overgrowth: Propionibacterium acnes (P. acnes), a type of bacteria that normally resides on the skin, can

proliferate in clogged pores and trigger inflammation, worsening acne lesions.

3. Inflammation: Inflammatory mediators released by the immune system in response to bacterial overgrowth and clogged pores contribute to redness, swelling, and pain associated with acne lesions.
4. Genetics: A family history of acne can increase the likelihood of developing the condition, suggesting a genetic predisposition to acne susceptibility.
5. Lifestyle Factors: Diet, stress, smoking, and certain medications can influence sebum production, inflammation, and skin cell turnover, impacting acne severity.

Types of Acne:

Acne can manifest in various forms, each with its unique characteristics and treatment approaches:

1. Comedonal Acne: Characterized by open (blackheads) and closed (whiteheads) comedones, comedonal acne involves clogged pores without significant inflammation.
2. Inflammatory Acne: Inflammatory acne presents with red, swollen papules, pustules, nodules, and cysts, indicating an inflammatory response to bacterial overgrowth.
3. Hormonal Acne: Hormonal fluctuations, particularly during puberty, menstruation, pregnancy, and menopause, can exacerbate acne by increasing sebum production and inflammation.
4. Adult-Onset Acne: Acne that persists into adulthood or develops later in life can be triggered by hormonal changes, stress, lifestyle factors, or underlying medical conditions.

Strategies for Managing Acne:

While acne can be frustrating and challenging to treat, a comprehensive approach that addresses underlying causes and incorporates targeted skincare treatments can help clear up troublesome skin and prevent future breakouts. Here are some effective strategies for managing acne:

1. Cleansing: Gentle cleansing twice daily with a mild, non-comedogenic cleanser helps remove excess oil, dirt, and impurities without stripping the skin's natural moisture barrier.
2. Exfoliation: Regular exfoliation with salicylic acid or alpha hydroxy acids (AHAs) helps unclog pores, remove dead skin cells, and promote cell turnover, reducing the risk of acne breakouts.
3. Topical Treatments: Over-the-counter and prescription treatments containing ingredients like benzoyl peroxide, retinoids, salicylic acid, and azelaic acid target acne-causing bacteria, reduce inflammation, and prevent new blemishes from forming.
4. Moisturization: Despite popular belief, moisturizing is essential for acne-prone skin to maintain hydration and prevent excess oil production. Choose lightweight, non-comedogenic moisturizers that won't clog pores.
5. Sun Protection: Protecting the skin from UV radiation with broad-spectrum sunscreen helps prevent post-inflammatory hyperpigmentation and reduces the risk of acne scarring.
6. Lifestyle Modifications: Adopting a healthy lifestyle that includes regular exercise, balanced nutrition, stress management, and adequate sleep can support overall skin health and reduce acne severity.
7. Professional Treatments: In-office procedures such as chemical peels, microdermabrasion, laser therapy, and corticosteroid injections may be recommended for severe or persistent acne that doesn't respond to conventional treatments.

11. BRIGHTENING TECHNIQUES

Fading Dark Spots and Hyperpigmentation

Achieving radiant skin isn't just about preventing acne or maintaining hydration; it's also about achieving an even, luminous complexion. Unfortunately, many of us struggle with hyperpigmentation, dark spots, and uneven skin tone, which can detract from our skin's natural beauty. In this chapter of "Radiant Skin: The Ultimate Guide to Boosting Your Complexion," we'll explore brightening techniques to effectively fade dark spots and hyperpigmentation, helping you achieve a clear, glowing complexion.

Understanding Hyperpigmentation:

Hyperpigmentation refers to the darkening of patches or areas of skin caused by excess melanin production. Melanin is the pigment responsible for giving our skin its color, and its production can be influenced by various factors, including sun exposure, hormonal changes, inflammation, and skin injuries. Common types of hyperpigmentation include:

1. Sunspots or Solar Lentigines: Also known as age spots or liver spots, sunspots are flat, brown spots that develop on sun-exposed areas of the skin, such as the face, hands, and arms, due to cumulative sun damage.

2. Post-Inflammatory Hyperpigmentation (PIH): PIH occurs as a result of inflammation or injury to the skin, such as acne, cuts, burns, or insect bites. Dark spots or patches may persist long after the initial injury has healed.

3. Melasma: Melasma is a common condition characterized by brown or grayish patches on the face, particularly on the cheeks, forehead, upper lip, and chin. Hormonal changes, such as pregnancy or hormonal therapy, can trigger melasma.

4. Freckles: Freckles are small, flat, brown spots that appear on sun-exposed areas of the skin, primarily in individuals with fair skin and a genetic predisposition to freckling.

Brightening Techniques:

While hyperpigmentation can be stubborn and challenging to treat, several brightening techniques can help fade dark spots and even out skin tone. It's essential to adopt a multi-faceted approach that addresses the underlying causes of hyperpigmentation and incorporates targeted treatments into your skincare routine. Here are some effective brightening techniques to consider:

1. Sun Protection: Preventing further sun damage is crucial for fading existing dark spots and preventing new ones from forming. Apply broad-spectrum sunscreen with SPF 30 or higher daily, even on cloudy days, and reapply every two hours or immediately after swimming or sweating.

2. Topical Treatments: Over-the-counter and prescription skincare products containing active ingredients such as hydroquinone, retinoids (vitamin A derivatives), vitamin C, niacinamide (vitamin B3), kojic acid, alpha hydroxy acids (AHAs), and azelaic acid can help fade dark spots, inhibit melanin production, and promote skin renewal.

3. Chemical Peels: Professional chemical peels using alpha and beta hydroxy acids, such as glycolic acid, salicylic acid, and lactic acid, exfoliate the skin's surface, fade hyperpigmentation, and stimulate collagen production for a brighter, more youthful complexion.

4. Laser Therapy: Various laser and light-based therapies, such as intense pulsed light (IPL), fractional lasers, and Q-switched lasers, target melanin in the skin to fade dark spots and improve overall skin tone. Laser treatments are particularly effective for stubborn or deep-seated hyperpigmentation.
5. Microneedling: Microneedling, also known as collagen induction therapy, involves using tiny needles to create micro-injuries in the skin, stimulating collagen production and enhancing the penetration of brightening serums and topical treatments.
6. Botanical Extracts: Natural ingredients such as licorice extract, bearberry extract, mulberry extract, green tea extract, and niacinamide have antioxidant and skin-brightening properties, helping to fade dark spots and improve overall skin tone without harsh side effects.

Developing a Brightening Skincare Routine:

To effectively fade dark spots and hyperpigmentation, it's essential to develop a customized skincare routine that addresses your specific concerns and incorporates targeted brightening treatments. Here's a step-by-step guide to brightening your complexion:

1. Cleanse: Start with a gentle cleanser to remove dirt, oil, and impurities from the skin without stripping its natural moisture barrier.
2. Tone: Use a gentle, alcohol-free toner to balance the skin's pH levels and prepare it for optimal absorption of brightening treatments.
3. Treat: Apply a targeted brightening serum or treatment containing active ingredients such as vitamin C, niacinamide, or hydroquinone to fade dark spots and even out skin tone.
4. Protect: Finish with a broad-spectrum sunscreen with SPF 30 or higher to protect the skin from further sun damage and prevent dark spots from worsening.
5. Hydrate: Moisturize the skin with a lightweight, non-comedogenic moisturizer to maintain hydration and support

skin barrier function.

Consistency is key when it comes to brightening treatments, and results may take time to become noticeable. It's essential to be patient and diligent with your skincare routine, and to avoid excessive sun exposure and harsh skincare products that can exacerbate hyperpigmentation. If you have stubborn or persistent dark spots, consider consulting a dermatologist or skincare professional for personalized treatment recommendations.

12. AGE-DEFYING SKINCARE

Turning Back the Clock on Wrinkles and Fine Lines

As we age, our skin undergoes various changes, including a decrease in collagen and elastin production, reduced cell turnover, and the formation of wrinkles and fine lines. While aging is a natural process, there are proactive steps we can take to minimize its visible effects and maintain a youthful, radiant complexion. In this chapter of "Radiant Skin: The Ultimate Guide to Boosting Your Complexion," we'll explore age-defying skincare techniques, including preventive measures, targeted treatments, and lifestyle adjustments, to help turn back the clock on wrinkles and fine lines.

Understanding the Aging Process:

Before delving into age-defying skincare techniques, it's essential to understand the underlying mechanisms of skin aging. Several factors contribute to the formation of wrinkles and fine lines:

1. Decreased Collagen and Elastin Production: Collagen and elastin are proteins responsible for maintaining the skin's structure, elasticity, and firmness. As we age, collagen and elastin production decreases, leading to sagging skin and the formation of wrinkles.

2. Reduced Hyaluronic Acid Levels: Hyaluronic acid is a naturally occurring substance that helps retain moisture in the skin, providing volume and plumpness. With age, hyaluronic acid levels decline, resulting in dryness and fine lines.
3. Oxidative Stress: Environmental factors such as UV radiation, pollution, and smoking generate free radicals in the skin, causing oxidative stress and accelerating the aging process.
4. Glycation: Glycation is a process in which sugar molecules bind to proteins like collagen and elastin, leading to the formation of advanced glycation end products (AGEs). AGEs contribute to skin stiffness, wrinkles, and loss of elasticity.
5. Muscle Movement: Repetitive facial expressions, such as smiling, squinting, and frowning, can lead to dynamic wrinkles, which become more prominent over time.

Age-Defying Skincare Techniques:

While we cannot stop the aging process entirely, we can adopt age-defying skincare techniques to minimize its visible effects and maintain a youthful appearance. Here are some effective strategies for turning back the clock on wrinkles and fine lines:

1. Sun Protection: Protecting the skin from UV radiation is crucial for preventing premature aging and reducing the formation of wrinkles and fine lines. Apply broad-spectrum sunscreen with SPF 30 or higher daily, even on cloudy days, and reapply every two hours or immediately after swimming or sweating.
2. Moisturization: Hydrating the skin with moisturizers containing humectants like hyaluronic acid and glycerin helps maintain moisture levels, plumpness, and elasticity, reducing the appearance of fine lines and wrinkles.
3. Retinoids: Retinoids, derivatives of vitamin A, are among the most effective anti-aging ingredients available. They stimulate collagen production, promote cell turnover, and improve skin texture, reducing the appearance of wrinkles, fine lines, and uneven pigmentation.

4. Antioxidants: Antioxidants such as vitamin C, vitamin E, and green tea extract neutralize free radicals, protect against oxidative stress, and help prevent collagen degradation and premature aging.
5. Peptides: Peptides are short chains of amino acids that stimulate collagen synthesis, improve skin elasticity, and reduce the appearance of wrinkles and fine lines.
6. Growth Factors: Growth factors are proteins that regulate cell growth, proliferation, and differentiation. Topical formulations containing growth factors can stimulate collagen production, improve skin texture, and reduce the signs of aging.
7. Hyaluronic Acid Fillers: Hyaluronic acid fillers are injectable treatments that add volume and plumpness to the skin, reducing the appearance of wrinkles and restoring youthful contours.
8. Chemical Peels: Professional chemical peels using alpha and beta hydroxy acids exfoliate the skin's surface, stimulate collagen production, and improve skin texture, reducing the appearance of wrinkles and fine lines.
9. Microneedling: Microneedling, also known as collagen induction therapy, involves using tiny needles to create micro-injuries in the skin, stimulating collagen production and improving skin texture and elasticity.
10. Botox and Dysport: Botulinum toxin injections, such as Botox and Dysport, temporarily relax facial muscles, reducing the appearance of dynamic wrinkles caused by repetitive facial expressions.

Developing an Age-Defying Skincare Routine:

To effectively combat wrinkles and fine lines, it's essential to develop a customized skincare routine tailored to your specific concerns and skin type. Here's a step-by-step guide to an age-defying skincare routine:

1. Cleanse: Start with a gentle cleanser to remove dirt, oil, and impurities from the skin without stripping its natural moisture barrier.

2. Tone: Use a toner containing antioxidants or hyaluronic acid to hydrate, balance, and prepare the skin for optimal absorption of age-defying treatments.
3. Treat: Apply targeted anti-aging serums or treatments containing retinoids, antioxidants, peptides, or growth factors to stimulate collagen production, improve skin texture, and reduce the appearance of wrinkles and fine lines.
4. Moisturize: Hydrate the skin with a rich, nourishing moisturizer containing ingredients like hyaluronic acid, ceramides, and antioxidants to lock in moisture, plumpness, and elasticity.
5. Protect: Finish with broad-spectrum sunscreen with SPF 30 or higher to shield the skin from UV radiation and prevent further photoaging and collagen degradation.
6. Special Treatments: Incorporate specialized treatments such as retinoid creams, antioxidant serums, or hyaluronic acid fillers into your skincare routine as needed, based on your skin concerns and goals.

13. HOLISTIC APPROACHES TO HEALTHY SKIN

Mind, Body, and Spirit

I n our quest for radiant skin, we often focus solely on external factors such as skincare products and treatments. However, true skin health encompasses more than just what meets the eye. Holistic approaches to healthy skin recognize the interconnectedness of the mind, body, and spirit, emphasizing the importance of nurturing our overall well-being to achieve a luminous complexion. In this chapter of "Radiant Skin: The Ultimate Guide to Boosting Your Complexion," we'll explore holistic approaches to healthy skin, incorporating nutrition, stress management, lifestyle habits, and mindfulness techniques to support skin health from within.

The Mind-Body Connection:

The mind-body connection refers to the link between our thoughts, emotions, and physical health. Studies have shown that stress, anxiety, and negative emotions can impact various physiological processes in the body, including skin health. Chronic stress, in particular, can trigger inflammatory responses, disrupt hormonal balance, and impair skin barrier function, leading to a variety of skin issues such as acne, eczema, psoriasis, and premature aging.

Conversely, cultivating positive emotions, practicing mindfulness, and adopting stress-reduction techniques can have profound benefits for skin health. When we take care of our mental and emotional well-being, our skin reflects that balance and vitality, glowing from within.

Nutrition for Healthy Skin:

The old adage "you are what you eat" holds true when it comes to skin health. A well-balanced diet rich in essential nutrients, vitamins, minerals, antioxidants, and omega-3 fatty acids can nourish the skin from the inside out, promoting cell renewal, collagen production, and overall skin vitality.

Key nutrients for healthy skin include:

1. Vitamin C: Vitamin C is a powerful antioxidant that protects the skin from free radical damage, promotes collagen synthesis, and brightens the complexion.
2. Vitamin E: Vitamin E helps protect the skin from UV damage, reduces inflammation, and supports skin barrier function.
3. Vitamin A: Vitamin A derivatives, such as retinoids, regulate cell turnover, stimulate collagen production, and improve skin texture and tone.
4. Omega-3 Fatty Acids: Omega-3 fatty acids found in fatty fish, flaxseeds, and walnuts help maintain skin hydration, reduce inflammation, and support skin barrier function.
5. Antioxidants: Antioxidants such as beta-carotene, lycopene, and polyphenols protect the skin from oxidative stress and UV damage, helping to prevent premature aging and improve skin texture.

Incorporating a variety of nutrient-dense foods into your diet, including fruits, vegetables, whole grains, lean proteins, and healthy fats, can provide the building blocks your skin needs to thrive.

Stress Management Techniques:

Chronic stress not only takes a toll on our mental and emotional well-being but also manifests physically in our skin. Incorporating stress management techniques into our daily routine can help reduce cortisol levels, promote relaxation, and improve overall skin health. Some effective stress management techniques include:

1. Mindfulness Meditation: Mindfulness meditation involves focusing on the present moment without judgment, helping to calm the mind, reduce stress, and promote emotional resilience.
2. Deep Breathing Exercises: Deep breathing exercises, such as diaphragmatic breathing or belly breathing, activate the body's relaxation response, lowering heart rate, blood pressure, and stress hormone levels.
3. Yoga: Yoga combines physical postures, breathwork, and meditation to promote relaxation, flexibility, and stress relief. Regular yoga practice has been shown to improve mood, reduce anxiety, and enhance overall well-being.
4. Nature Walks: Spending time in nature, whether it's a walk in the park, a hike in the mountains, or a stroll on the beach, can have a calming effect on the mind and body, reducing stress and promoting a sense of well-being.
5. Creative Expression: Engaging in creative activities such as painting, writing, music, or crafting allows for self-expression, stress relief, and a sense of accomplishment.

Lifestyle Habits for Healthy Skin:

In addition to nutrition and stress management, certain lifestyle habits can support skin health and promote a radiant complexion:

1. Adequate Sleep: Quality sleep is essential for skin repair and regeneration. Aim for 7-9 hours of uninterrupted sleep per night to allow your skin to rest and rejuvenate.
2. Hydration: Drinking an adequate amount of water daily helps maintain skin hydration, flush out toxins, and support overall skin health. Aim for at least 8 glasses of water per day, or more if you're physically active or live in a hot climate.
3. Regular Exercise: Exercise improves blood circulation, reduces stress, and promotes a healthy glow. Aim for at least 30 minutes

of moderate-intensity exercise most days of the week to reap the benefits for your skin and overall well-being.

4. Skincare Routine: Establishing a consistent skincare routine tailored to your skin type and concerns is essential for maintaining healthy skin. Cleanse, tone, treat, moisturize, and protect your skin daily to keep it looking its best.

5. Sun Protection: Protecting your skin from UV radiation is crucial for preventing premature aging, sun damage, and skin cancer. Wear broad-spectrum sunscreen with SPF 30 or higher daily, seek shade, and wear protective clothing and sunglasses when outdoors.

14. EATING FOR RADIANCE

Nutrition Tips for Glowing Skin

W hen it comes to achieving radiant skin, skincare products and routines play a significant role. However, the foundation of healthy, glowing skin begins from within. What you eat can have a profound impact on the health and appearance of your skin. In this chapter of "Radiant Skin: The Ultimate Guide to Boosting Your Complexion," we'll explore the relationship between nutrition and skin health, and provide practical tips and guidelines for eating your way to radiant, glowing skin.

The Link Between Nutrition and Skin Health:

The old adage "you are what you eat" holds true when it comes to skin health. The foods you consume can influence various skin parameters, including hydration, elasticity, clarity, and overall radiance. Here's how nutrition impacts skin health:

1. Hydration: Drinking an adequate amount of water is essential for maintaining skin hydration. Dehydration can lead to dry, dull-looking skin, whereas proper hydration promotes a plump, radiant complexion.

2. Nutrient Intake: Vitamins, minerals, and antioxidants found in fruits, vegetables, and other nutrient-dense foods play vital roles in skin health. These nutrients support collagen production,

protect against oxidative stress, and promote skin repair and renewal.

3. Inflammation: Certain foods, such as sugary, processed, and fried foods, can promote inflammation in the body, leading to skin conditions like acne, eczema, and psoriasis. Consuming anti-inflammatory foods helps calm inflammation and promote clear, healthy skin.

4. Glycemic Index: Foods with a high glycemic index (GI), such as refined carbohydrates and sugary snacks, can spike blood sugar levels and contribute to acne breakouts and premature aging. Choosing low-GI foods helps maintain stable blood sugar levels and supports skin health.

Nutrition Tips for Glowing Skin:

To optimize your diet for radiant, glowing skin, consider incorporating the following nutrition tips into your daily routine:

1. Load Up on Fruits and Vegetables: Fruits and vegetables are packed with vitamins, minerals, and antioxidants that nourish the skin from the inside out. Aim to include a variety of colorful fruits and vegetables in your diet, such as berries, citrus fruits, leafy greens, carrots, and bell peppers.

2. Choose Healthy Fats: Omega-3 fatty acids found in fatty fish, walnuts, flaxseeds, and chia seeds help maintain skin hydration, reduce inflammation, and support skin barrier function. Incorporate sources of healthy fats into your diet regularly for supple, glowing skin.

3. Stay Hydrated: Drinking plenty of water throughout the day is essential for maintaining skin hydration and promoting a radiant complexion. Aim to consume at least eight glasses of water daily, and hydrate with herbal teas, infused water, and hydrating foods like cucumbers and watermelon.

4. Opt for Whole Grains: Choose whole grains such as oats, quinoa, brown rice, and barley over refined grains to support stable blood sugar levels and reduce the risk of acne breakouts and premature aging.

5. Limit Added Sugars: Minimize your intake of added sugars found in sugary snacks, desserts, and sweetened beverages, as they can promote inflammation, glycation, and skin aging. Instead, satisfy your sweet tooth with naturally sweet foods like fresh fruit or small amounts of dark chocolate.
6. Include Lean Proteins: Protein is essential for skin repair and renewal, collagen synthesis, and maintaining skin elasticity. Incorporate lean protein sources such as poultry, fish, tofu, legumes, and nuts into your meals to support healthy, radiant skin.
7. Consume Antioxidant-Rich Foods: Antioxidant-rich foods such as berries, dark leafy greens, nuts, seeds, and green tea help neutralize free radicals, protect against oxidative stress, and promote youthful, glowing skin.
8. Supplement Wisely: While a balanced diet should provide most of the nutrients your skin needs, certain supplements may benefit skin health, such as vitamin C, vitamin E, zinc, and collagen peptides. Consult with a healthcare professional before adding supplements to your regimen.

The Role of Skincare in Conjunction with Nutrition:

While nutrition plays a significant role in skin health, it's essential to complement your dietary efforts with a proper skincare routine. Cleansing, moisturizing, exfoliating, and protecting your skin from environmental stressors are essential for maintaining skin health and optimizing the benefits of a nutritious diet. Additionally, incorporating topical skincare products containing vitamins, antioxidants, and hydrating ingredients can further support radiant, glowing skin.

15. DIY SKINCARE RECIPES

Natural Remedies for a Luxurious Glow

In today's fast-paced world, the beauty industry bombards us with countless skincare products promising radiant, flawless skin. While these products can be effective, they often come with a hefty price tag and a list of synthetic ingredients that may not align with everyone's preferences. Fortunately, nature has provided us with an abundance of ingredients that offer skincare benefits without the harmful chemicals. In this chapter of "Radiant Skin: The Ultimate Guide to Boosting Your Complexion," we'll explore DIY skincare recipes using natural ingredients to achieve a luxurious glow from the comfort of your own home.

Why DIY Skincare?

DIY skincare offers several benefits beyond just saving money. By creating your own skincare products, you have full control over the ingredients used, ensuring they're fresh, natural, and tailored to your specific skin concerns. Additionally, DIY skincare allows you to experiment with different formulations and customize your products to suit your preferences, whether it's adding fragrance, adjusting consistency, or targeting specific issues like acne, dryness, or hyperpigmentation. Plus, crafting your skincare products can be a fun and rewarding experience that fosters a deeper connection with your skin and overall well-being.

Essential Ingredients for DIY Skincare:

Before diving into specific recipes, let's explore some essential ingredients commonly used in DIY skincare and their benefits:

1. Carrier Oils: Carrier oils are natural plant-based oils used as a base for skincare formulations. They provide hydration, nourishment, and essential fatty acids to the skin. Popular carrier oils include jojoba oil, sweet almond oil, coconut oil, argan oil, and rosehip seed oil.
2. Essential Oils: Essential oils are highly concentrated plant extracts prized for their therapeutic properties and aromatic fragrance. When used in skincare, they can offer a range of benefits, from soothing inflammation to promoting relaxation. Some popular essential oils for skincare include lavender, tea tree, rosemary, frankincense, and chamomile.
3. Natural Butters: Natural butters, such as shea butter, cocoa butter, and mango butter, are rich in vitamins, antioxidants, and fatty acids that nourish and moisturize the skin. They provide emollient properties and help improve skin elasticity and suppleness.
4. Exfoliants: Exfoliants help remove dead skin cells, unclog pores, and promote cell turnover, revealing smoother, brighter skin underneath. Common natural exfoliants include sugar, salt, coffee grounds, oatmeal, and ground nuts or seeds.
5. Botanical Extracts: Botanical extracts are concentrated plant extracts derived from flowers, herbs, fruits, and vegetables. They offer a range of skincare benefits, including antioxidant protection, anti-inflammatory properties, and skin conditioning. Examples include green tea extract, calendula extract, aloe vera gel, and witch hazel extract.

Now that we've covered the essential ingredients let's dive into some DIY skincare recipes for achieving a luxurious glow:

1. Hydrating Facial Oil:

Ingredients:

- 1 tablespoon jojoba oil
- 1 tablespoon rosehip seed oil
- 5 drops lavender essential oil
- 3 drops frankincense essential oil
- 2 drops geranium essential oil

Instructions:

1. In a small glass dropper bottle, combine the jojoba oil and rosehip seed oil.
2. Add the lavender, frankincense, and geranium essential oils to the carrier oils.
3. Secure the lid and shake the bottle gently to mix the ingredients thoroughly.
4. To use, apply a few drops of the facial oil to clean, damp skin and massage gently in upward circular motions. Allow the oil to absorb fully before applying additional skincare products or makeup.
5. Store the facial oil in a cool, dark place away from direct sunlight.

Benefits: This hydrating facial oil combines nourishing carrier oils with essential oils known for their skin-soothing and rejuvenating properties. Jojoba oil and rosehip seed oil provide intense hydration and deliver essential fatty acids and vitamins to the skin, while lavender, frankincense, and geranium essential oils promote relaxation, reduce inflammation, and improve skin tone and texture.

2. Soothing Oatmeal Face Mask:

Ingredients:

- 2 tablespoons finely ground oatmeal
- 1 tablespoon plain yogurt
- 1 teaspoon honey
- 1 teaspoon aloe vera gel

Instructions:

1. In a small bowl, combine the finely ground oatmeal, plain yogurt, honey, and aloe vera gel.
2. Stir the ingredients together until you achieve a smooth, uniform paste.
3. Apply the mask to clean, dry skin, avoiding the eye area.
4. Leave the mask on for 10-15 minutes to allow the ingredients to work their magic.
5. Rinse the mask off thoroughly with warm water, then pat the skin dry with a clean towel.
6. Follow up with your favorite moisturizer or facial oil to lock in hydration.

Benefits: This soothing oatmeal face mask is perfect for calming irritated or sensitive skin and providing gentle exfoliation. Oatmeal helps soothe inflammation and redness while gently removing dead skin cells, revealing smoother, more radiant skin underneath. Yogurt and honey offer additional hydration and nourishment, while aloe vera gel provides cooling relief and helps repair and rejuvenate the skin.

3. Brightening Turmeric Face Scrub:

Ingredients:

- 1 tablespoon coconut oil
- 1 tablespoon finely ground turmeric
- 1 tablespoon granulated sugar
- 1 teaspoon lemon juice

Instructions:

1. In a small bowl, melt the coconut oil until it's in liquid form.
2. Add the finely ground turmeric, granulated sugar, and lemon juice to the melted coconut oil.
3. Stir the ingredients together until you achieve a thick paste-like consistency.
4. Gently massage the scrub onto damp skin using circular motions, focusing on areas of concern such as dark spots or

hyperpigmentation.

5. Allow the scrub to sit on the skin for a few minutes to allow the ingredients to penetrate.
6. Rinse the scrub off thoroughly with warm water, then pat the skin dry with a clean towel.
7. Follow up with a moisturizer or facial oil to replenish hydration.

Benefits: This brightening turmeric face scrub harnesses the antioxidant and anti-inflammatory properties of turmeric to fade dark spots, even out skin tone, and promote a radiant complexion. Coconut oil provides moisturization and helps soothe and soften the skin, while granulated sugar offers gentle exfoliation to slough away dead skin cells and reveal brighter, smoother skin. Lemon juice contains natural alpha hydroxy acids (AHAs) that exfoliate the skin and promote cell turnover for a more youthful appearance.

4. Refreshing Cucumber Eye Gel:

Ingredients:

- 1/2 cucumber, peeled and grated
- 1 tablespoon aloe vera gel
- 1 tablespoon rose water

Instructions:

1. Place the grated cucumber in a fine-mesh sieve or cheesecloth and squeeze out the juice into a clean bowl.
2. Add the aloe vera gel and rose water to the cucumber juice.
3. Stir the ingredients together until well combined.
4. Transfer the mixture to a clean, airtight container and store it in the refrigerator for up to one week.
5. To use, apply a small amount of the cucumber eye gel to the under-eye area using gentle tapping motions.
6. Allow the gel to absorb fully into the skin, then follow up with your favorite eye cream or moisturizer.

Benefits: This refreshing cucumber eye gel is perfect for reducing puffiness, dark circles, and fatigue around the eyes. Cucumber contains antioxidants and anti-inflammatory properties that soothe and depuff the delicate under-eye area, while aloe vera gel provides hydration and helps improve skin elasticity. Rose water offers additional soothing and toning benefits, leaving the skin feeling refreshed and rejuvenated.

5. Nourishing Avocado Hair Mask:

Ingredients:

- 1 ripe avocado, mashed
- 1 tablespoon coconut oil
- 1 tablespoon honey
- 1 tablespoon plain yogurt

Instructions:

1. In a small bowl, combine the mashed avocado, coconut oil, honey, and plain yogurt.
2. Stir the ingredients together until you achieve a smooth, creamy consistency.
3. Apply the hair mask to clean, damp hair, focusing on the lengths and ends.
4. Massage the mask into the hair and scalp, ensuring even distribution.
5. Cover your hair with a shower cap or towel and leave the mask on for 30 minutes to an hour to allow the ingredients to penetrate.
6. Rinse the mask out thoroughly with warm water, then shampoo and condition your hair as usual.

Benefits: This nourishing avocado hair mask is packed with vitamins, minerals, and fatty acids that moisturize, strengthen, and revitalize dry, damaged hair. Avocado provides essential nutrients and hydration to the hair and scalp, while coconut oil helps repair and protect against environmental damage. Honey and yogurt offer additional nourishment and shine, leaving your hair soft, smooth, and lustrous.

16.MAKEUP TIPS AND TRICKS

Enhancing Your Complexion with Cosmetics

Makeup has the power to enhance our natural beauty, boost our confidence, and create a flawless complexion. Whether you're looking to even out your skin tone, camouflage imperfections, or add a touch of radiance, mastering the art of makeup application can help you achieve the glowing complexion of your dreams. In this chapter of "Radiant Skin: The Ultimate Guide to Boosting Your Complexion," we'll explore makeup tips and tricks for enhancing your complexion, from foundation selection to highlighting and contouring techniques.

Prepping Your Canvas:

Before applying makeup, it's essential to start with a clean, well-hydrated canvas. Proper skincare, including cleansing, exfoliating, moisturizing, and sun protection, lays the foundation for flawless makeup application. Here are some skincare tips to ensure your complexion is primed and ready for makeup:

1. Cleansing: Begin by cleansing your face with a gentle, hydrating cleanser to remove dirt, oil, and impurities without stripping the skin's natural moisture barrier.
2. Exfoliating: Exfoliate your skin regularly to slough off dead skin cells and reveal a smoother, more radiant complexion.

Choose a chemical exfoliant containing alpha or beta hydroxy acids for gentle, effective exfoliation.

3. Moisturizing: Hydrate your skin with a lightweight, non-comedogenic moisturizer to replenish moisture, plumpness, and elasticity. Allow the moisturizer to absorb fully before applying makeup.

4. Sun Protection: Protect your skin from harmful UV rays by applying broad-spectrum sunscreen with SPF 30 or higher daily, even on cloudy days. Opt for a lightweight, oil-free formula that won't feel heavy or greasy under makeup.

Choosing the Right Foundation:

Foundation serves as the base for your makeup look, providing coverage, evening out skin tone, and creating a smooth canvas for additional makeup products. Finding the perfect foundation match for your skin type and concerns is essential for achieving a flawless complexion. Here's how to choose the right foundation for your skin:

1. Determine Your Skin Type: Consider whether you have dry, oily, combination, or sensitive skin, as this will influence the type of foundation that works best for you.

2. Choose Your Coverage Level: Decide whether you prefer light, medium, or full coverage foundation based on your desired level of coverage and the imperfections you want to conceal.

3. Match Your Undertone: Determine whether your skin has warm, cool, or neutral undertones to find a foundation shade that complements your natural skin tone.

4. Test Shades: Test foundation shades on your jawline or neck to find the closest match to your skin tone. Natural light is best for determining an accurate shade match.

5. Consider Formulation: Choose a foundation formulation that suits your skin type and preferences, whether it's liquid, cream, powder, or mineral foundation.

Application Techniques:

Once you've selected the perfect foundation, it's time to apply it to your skin for a flawless finish. Here are some application techniques to achieve a seamless, natural-looking complexion:

1. Use a Makeup Primer: Apply a makeup primer to your skin before foundation to create a smooth, even base and extend the wear of your makeup. Choose a primer that addresses your specific concerns, such as blurring pores, hydrating dry skin, or controlling oil.
2. Apply Foundation Sparingly: Start with a small amount of foundation and build up coverage gradually as needed. Use a makeup sponge, brush, or your fingertips to blend the foundation seamlessly into your skin, focusing on areas that require extra coverage.
3. Blend Well: Blend foundation thoroughly along the jawline, hairline, and neck to avoid harsh lines or demarcation. Take your time to ensure a seamless transition between your natural skin and the foundation.
4. Set with Powder: Set your foundation with a translucent or tinted setting powder to lock it in place and reduce shine. Use a fluffy brush to dust powder lightly over the face, concentrating on areas prone to oiliness.

Concealing Imperfections:

Even with foundation, you may still have imperfections such as dark circles, blemishes, or redness that require additional coverage. Concealer is a versatile makeup product that can camouflage these imperfections and create a flawless complexion. Here's how to use concealer effectively:

1. Choose the Right Shade: Select a concealer shade that matches your foundation or is slightly lighter to brighten and highlight the under-eye area.
2. Target Specific Areas: Apply concealer sparingly to areas that need extra coverage, such as under-eye circles, blemishes, redness, or dark spots.
3. Blend with Fingertips or Brush: Use your fingertips or a small concealer brush to blend the concealer seamlessly into the skin,

tapping gently to ensure smooth, even coverage.

4. Set with Powder: Set your concealer with a light dusting of translucent setting powder to prevent creasing and ensure long-lasting wear.

Enhancing Your Glow:

Once you've perfected your complexion with foundation and concealer, it's time to add dimension and radiance to your skin with highlighting and contouring techniques. Highlighter and contour products help define your features, create depth, and enhance your natural bone structure. Here's how to master highlighting and contouring:

1. Highlight: Apply a cream or powder highlighter to the high points of your face, including the tops of your cheekbones, brow bones, bridge of the nose, and cupid's bow. Use a light hand and blend well for a subtle, luminous glow.
2. Contour: Use a matte bronzer or contour powder to sculpt and define your facial features. Apply the contour product to the hollows of your cheeks, along the jawline, and the sides of the nose to create shadows and add dimension.
3. Blend Thoroughly: Blend the highlighter and contour products seamlessly into the skin using a makeup sponge or blending brush. Take your time to ensure a natural-looking finish without harsh lines or streaks.
4. Set with Setting Spray: Set your makeup with a setting spray to lock everything in place and enhance the longevity of your makeup look. Choose a setting spray that offers a dewy or matte finish, depending on your preference.

Adding the Finishing Touches:

To complete your makeup look and enhance your complexion further, consider adding the following finishing touches:

1. Blush: Apply a natural-looking blush to the apples of your cheeks for a healthy flush of color. Choose a blush shade that

complements your skin tone and adds warmth and vitality to your complexion.

2. Lip Color: Select a lip color that enhances your complexion and ties your makeup look together. Whether you prefer a bold lip or a subtle nude, choose a lip color that makes you feel confident and radiant.

3. Setting Powder: If necessary, touch up your makeup throughout the day with a translucent setting powder to absorb excess oil and maintain a fresh, matte finish.

4. Setting Spray: Finish your makeup look with a final spritz of setting spray to lock in your makeup and keep it looking flawless all day long.

17.STRESS MANAGEMENT FOR BETTER SKIN

Finding Balance in a Busy World

In today's fast-paced world, stress has become an unavoidable part of daily life for many people. Whether it's due to work pressures, personal responsibilities, or societal expectations, chronic stress can take a toll on our physical, mental, and emotional well-being. One area where stress often manifests is in our skin. From breakouts and dullness to premature aging and inflammation, stress can wreak havoc on our complexion, leaving us feeling less than radiant. In this chapter of "Radiant Skin: The Ultimate Guide to Boosting Your Complexion," we'll explore the connection between stress and skin health and discuss effective strategies for managing stress to achieve a clear, glowing complexion. Understanding the Stress-Skin Connection:

The relationship between stress and skin health is complex and multifaceted. When we experience stress, our bodies release hormones like cortisol and adrenaline as part of the "fight or flight" response. While these hormones are essential for survival in acute stress situations, chronic stress can lead to imbalances in hormone levels, inflammation, and oxidative damage, all of which can negatively impact our skin. Here are some ways in which stress can affect our complexion:

1. Acne and Breakouts: Stress triggers the release of cortisol, which can increase sebum production and inflammation in the skin, leading to acne breakouts and exacerbating existing skin conditions like acne vulgaris, eczema, and psoriasis.
2. Dullness and Fatigue: Chronic stress can disrupt the skin's natural barrier function, leading to dehydration, dullness, and a lackluster complexion. Stress-induced sleep disturbances and fatigue can also contribute to dark circles and under-eye puffiness, making the skin appear tired and worn out.
3. Premature Aging: Prolonged exposure to stress hormones like cortisol can accelerate the aging process by promoting collagen breakdown, elastin degradation, and oxidative stress, leading to wrinkles, fine lines, and sagging skin.
4. Sensitivity and Irritation: Stress can weaken the skin's natural defense mechanisms, making it more susceptible to environmental aggressors like pollution, UV radiation, and harsh skincare products. This can result in increased skin sensitivity, redness, and irritation.
5. Delayed Healing: Stress impairs the skin's ability to repair and regenerate itself, slowing down the healing process for wounds, blemishes, and other skin injuries.

Managing Stress for Better Skin:

While we may not be able to eliminate stress entirely from our lives, we can adopt effective strategies for managing stress and minimizing its impact on our skin. Here are some stress management techniques to promote better skin health and overall well-being:

1. Practice Mindfulness and Meditation: Mindfulness practices like meditation, deep breathing, and progressive muscle relaxation can help calm the mind, reduce stress levels, and promote a sense of inner peace and tranquility. Incorporate mindfulness exercises into your daily routine to manage stress more effectively and cultivate a positive mindset.
2. Prioritize Self-Care: Make self-care a priority by carving out time for activities that nourish your body, mind, and soul.

Whether it's taking a long bath, going for a nature walk, practicing yoga, or indulging in your favorite hobbies, self-care rituals can help reduce stress, boost mood, and improve skin health.

3. Get Adequate Sleep: Aim for 7-9 hours of quality sleep per night to allow your body and skin to rest, repair, and regenerate. Establish a relaxing bedtime routine, create a comfortable sleep environment, and avoid caffeine, electronic devices, and stimulating activities before bedtime to promote better sleep quality.

4. Exercise Regularly: Engage in regular physical activity to reduce stress, increase endorphin levels, and improve circulation, which can benefit skin health by delivering oxygen and nutrients to the skin cells and promoting a healthy glow. Choose activities you enjoy, whether it's yoga, swimming, dancing, or jogging, and aim for at least 30 minutes of moderate exercise most days of the week.

5. Eat a Balanced Diet: Fuel your body with nutrient-rich foods that support skin health from the inside out. Incorporate a variety of fruits, vegetables, whole grains, lean proteins, and healthy fats into your diet to provide essential vitamins, minerals, antioxidants, and omega-3 fatty acids that promote healthy skin function and combat the effects of stress and inflammation.

6. Stay Hydrated: Drink plenty of water throughout the day to stay hydrated and support optimal skin hydration and elasticity. Limit consumption of dehydrating beverages like alcohol and caffeine, which can exacerbate stress and deplete the skin of moisture.

7. Establish Boundaries: Set boundaries and learn to say no to excessive demands on your time, energy, and resources. Prioritize tasks, delegate responsibilities, and avoid overcommitting yourself to prevent feelings of overwhelm and burnout.

8. Seek Support: Reach out to friends, family members, or a mental health professional for support and guidance during

stressful times. Talking about your feelings, seeking advice, and receiving emotional support can help alleviate stress and promote resilience.

9. Practice Gratitude: Cultivate an attitude of gratitude by focusing on the positive aspects of your life and expressing appreciation for the blessings you have. Keep a gratitude journal, write down three things you're grateful for each day, or take a moment to savor small moments of joy and beauty in your everyday life.

10. Limit Stressors: Identify sources of stress in your life and take proactive steps to minimize or eliminate them where possible. This may involve setting boundaries with toxic relationships, reducing exposure to negative news or social media, simplifying your schedule, or seeking professional help for chronic stressors like work-related stress or financial concerns.

18. YOUR SKINCARE ROUTINE

Customizing a Regimen for Your Unique Needs

Achieving radiant, glowing skin is a journey that requires dedication, patience, and a tailored skincare routine designed to address your unique needs and concerns. In this final chapter of "Radiant Skin: The Ultimate Guide to Boosting Your Complexion," we'll explore the importance of customizing a skincare regimen that works for you and provide expert insights, tips, and recommendations for creating a personalized routine that promotes optimal skin health and vitality. Understanding Your Skin:

Before diving into building your skincare routine, it's essential to understand your skin type, concerns, and goals. Skin types can vary widely from person to person and may include categories such as dry, oily, combination, sensitive, or normal. Additionally, you may have specific skin concerns or conditions that you'd like to address, such as acne, aging, hyperpigmentation, dehydration, or sensitivity. By identifying your skin type and concerns, you can choose products and ingredients that are best suited to your individual needs and preferences.

Building Your Skincare Routine:

A well-rounded skincare routine typically consists of several essential steps designed to cleanse, exfoliate, hydrate, protect, and treat the skin. While the specific products and techniques may vary depending on your skin type and concerns, the following steps form the foundation of a basic skincare routine:

1. Cleansing: Cleansing is the first step in any skincare routine and is essential for removing dirt, oil, makeup, and impurities from the skin. Choose a gentle, pH-balanced cleanser suited to your skin type, and cleanse your face morning and night to keep your skin clean and refreshed.

2. Exfoliation: Exfoliation helps remove dead skin cells, unclog pores, and promote cell turnover, resulting in smoother, brighter skin. Incorporate a chemical or physical exfoliant into your routine 2-3 times per week, depending on your skin's tolerance and sensitivity level.

3. Toning: Toners help balance the skin's pH, tighten pores, and prepare the skin for subsequent skincare steps. Choose a hydrating, alcohol-free toner that suits your skin type and concerns, and apply it after cleansing to refresh and rebalance your skin.

4. Treatment: Treatments are targeted products designed to address specific skin concerns, such as acne, aging, hyperpigmentation, or dehydration. Incorporate treatment products like serums, essences, ampoules, or spot treatments into your routine to address your unique skincare needs.

5. Hydration: Hydration is crucial for maintaining healthy, plump, and supple skin. Choose a lightweight, hydrating moisturizer or facial oil suited to your skin type and concerns, and apply it morning and night to lock in moisture and nourish your skin.

6. Sun Protection: Sunscreen is a non-negotiable step in any skincare routine, regardless of your skin type or concerns. Apply a broad-spectrum sunscreen with SPF 30 or higher every morning to protect your skin from the harmful effects of UV radiation and prevent premature aging, sun damage, and skin cancer.

Customizing Your Skincare Routine:

Once you've established the basic steps of your skincare routine, it's time to customize it to address your unique needs and concerns. Here are some tips for customizing your skincare routine:

1. Identify Your Priorities: Determine the primary goals and concerns you'd like to address with your skincare routine, whether it's reducing acne breakouts, minimizing fine lines and wrinkles, fading dark spots, or improving hydration and texture.

2. Choose Targeted Products: Select skincare products and ingredients that target your specific concerns and goals. Look for active ingredients like retinol, vitamin C, niacinamide, hyaluronic acid, AHAs, BHAs, peptides, antioxidants, and botanical extracts that address your unique skincare needs.

3. Layer Products Wisely: Pay attention to the order and frequency of application when layering skincare products in your routine. Start with lightweight, water-based products and gradually layer thicker, oil-based products on top to ensure optimal absorption and efficacy.

4. Listen to Your Skin: Pay attention to how your skin responds to different products and ingredients, and adjust your skincare routine accordingly. If you experience irritation, sensitivity, or breakouts, scale back on active ingredients or switch to gentler formulations to prevent further damage.

5. Be Consistent: Consistency is key to seeing results with your skincare routine. Stick to your regimen consistently, morning and night, and give your skin time to adjust and respond to the products you're using. It may take several weeks or months to see significant improvements, so be patient and stay committed to your skincare journey.

6. Seek Professional Advice: If you're unsure about which products or ingredients are best for your skin type and concerns, consider seeking advice from a dermatologist or skincare professional. They can assess your skin, provide personalized recommendations, and help you create a tailored skincare routine that addresses your specific needs.

Sample Skincare Routine:

To help you get started, here's a sample skincare routine tailored to different skin types and concerns:

Morning Routine:

1. Cleanse with a gentle foaming cleanser.
2. Apply a hydrating toner to balance and refresh the skin.
3. Follow with a vitamin C serum to brighten and protect against environmental damage.
4. Apply a lightweight moisturizer or facial oil to hydrate and nourish the skin.
5. Finish with a broad-spectrum sunscreen with SPF 30 or higher.

Evening Routine:

1. Double cleanse to remove makeup, sunscreen, and impurities.
2. Exfoliate with a gentle chemical exfoliant (2-3 times per week).
3. Apply a retinol or peptide serum to target signs of aging.
4. Follow with a hydrating moisturizer or facial oil to replenish moisture.
5. Use an overnight mask or treatment as needed for additional hydration or repair.

CONCLUSION

Customizing a skincare routine that addresses your unique needs and concerns is essential for achieving radiant, healthy skin. By understanding your skin type, identifying your priorities, and choosing targeted products and ingredients, you can create a personalized skincare regimen that promotes optimal skin health and vitality. Whether you're dealing with acne, aging, hyperpigmentation, or sensitivity, there's a skincare routine tailored to your individual needs. Remember to be patient, consistent, and attentive to your skin's response as you embark on your skincare journey. With dedication, knowledge, and the right products, you can unlock the secrets to radiant, glowing skin and enjoy the confidence and beauty that comes with it.

Thank you for joining us on this journey through "Radiant Skin: The Ultimate Guide to Boosting Your Complexion." We hope you've found valuable insights, tips, and recommendations to enhance your skin's radiance and beauty naturally. May your skincare routine be a source of joy, self-care, and empowerment as you continue on your path to radiant, glowing skin.

Wishing you health, happiness, and radiant beauty now and always.

Milton Keynes UK
Ingram Content Group UK Ltd.
UKHW052302290324
440241UK00012B/416